The Essential Low Sodium Recipe Book

Tasty and Affordable Low Sodium Recipes to Start Your Day with the Right Foot

Jennifer Loyel

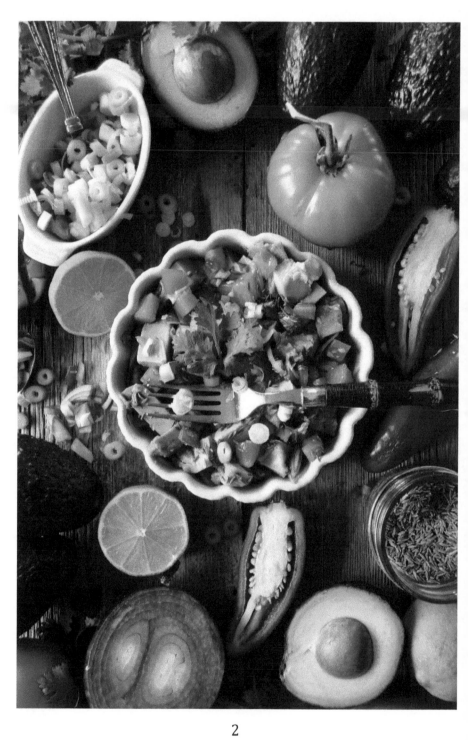

professional advice. The content within this book has been derived from various sources. Please consult a licensed professional before attempting any techniques outlined in this book.

By reading this document, the reader agrees that under no circumstances is the author responsible for any losses, direct or indirect, which are incurred as a result of the use of information contained within this document, including, but not limited to, — errors, omissions, or inaccuracies.

Table of Contents

7

Maple Turkey Sausage

Servings: 4

Ingredients:

- 1 pound lean ground turkey
- 1 tablespoon maple syrup
- 1/4 teaspoon freshly ground black pepper
- 1/8 teaspoon mustard powder
- 1/8 teaspoon ground cloves
- 1/8 teaspoon ground sage
- Pinch ground cinnamon
- Pinch ground allspice
- Pinch ground mace
- Optional: 1/4 teaspoon natural maple flavoring

Directions:

1. Mix together all the ingredients in a bowl. Cover and refrigerate overnight.
2. Shape the mixture into 4 flat patties. Cook over medium heat in a medium nonstick skillet or grill pan for 3 minutes on each side or until a food thermometer registers 165°F.

Nutrition Info: (Per Serving):Calories: 167; Total Fat: 7 g; Saturated Fat: 0 g; Cholesterol: 65 mg; Protein:

22 g; Sodium: 81 mg; Potassium: 14 mg; Fiber: 0 g; Carbohydrates: 3 g; Sugar: 3 g

Waffles

Servings: 2

Ingredients:

- 1 cup (110 g) all-purpose flour
- 1 teaspoon sodium-free baking powder
- 1 teaspoon sugar
- 1 egg
- ¾ cup (175 ml) skim milk
- 1 tablespoon (14 g) unsalted butter, melted

Directions:

1. Mix together dry ingredients. Combine egg, milk, and melted butter. Add to dry ingredients, mixing until just blended. Do not overbeat. Bake according to waffle iron directions.

Nutrition Info: (Per Serving): 113 g water; 369 calories (23% from fat, 15% from protein, 62% from carb); 14 g protein; 9 g total fat; 5 g saturated fat; 3 g monounsaturated fat; 1 g polyunsaturated fat; 56 g carb; 2 g fiber; 2 g sugar; 267 mg calcium; 4 mg iron; 99 mg sodium; 528 mg potassium; 506 IU vitamin A; 1 mg vitamin C; 140 mg cholesterol

Apple Potato Pancakes

Servings: 4

Ingredients:

- 1/2 cup potato flakes
- 11/2 cups boiling water
- 4 large eggs
- 2 teaspoons granulated sugar
- 1/2 teaspoon ground cinnamon
- 1 cup peeled and grated Granny Smith apple
- 1/4 cup chopped pecans
- Optional: Plain nonfat yogurt, sour cream, or applesauce

Directions:

1. To prepare the potatoes, add potato flakes to a large bowl. Gradually pour the boiling water over the potato flakes, whisking continuously to mix and whip.
2. In small bowl, beat together the eggs, sugar, and cinnamon. Beat into the potatoes. Fold in the grated apple and chopped pecans.
3. Heat a nonstick skillet or griddle treated with nonstick spray over medium heat. (If using an

electric griddle, preheat to 350°F–380°F.) Cook the pancakes on both sides until golden brown. Serve hot—plain or topped with plain nonfat yogurt, sour cream, or applesauce.

Nutrition Info: (Per Serving):Calories: 176; Total Fat: 10 g; Saturated Fat: 2 g; Cholesterol: 211 mg; Protein: 7 g; Sodium: 78 mg; Potassium: 209 mg; Fiber: 1 g; Carbohydrates: 13 g; Sugar: 5 g

Buckwheat Pancakes

Servings: 4

Ingredients:

- 1/2 cup whole-wheat flour
- 1/2 cup unbleached all-purpose flour
- 1/2 cup buckwheat flour
- 1/2 teaspoon baking powder
- 1 large egg, separated
- 3 tablespoons apple juice concentrate
- 1 tablespoon lemon juice
- 11/4–11/2 cups skim milk

Directions:

1. Sift the flours and baking powder together in a large bowl.

2. Combine the egg yolk, apple juice concentrate, lemon juice, and 1 cup of the skim milk in a small bowl. Add the milk mixture to the dry ingredients and mix well, but do not overmix. Add the remaining milk if necessary to reach your desired consistency.

3. In small bowl, beat the egg white until stiff peaks form. Fold into the batter until just combined.

4.   Cook the pancakes, using 1/4 cup measure for each one, in a nonstick skillet or on a griddle treated with nonstick spray over medium heat until the top of the pancake bubbles and the edges begin to look dry. Flip pancakes using a spatula; cook for 1–2 minutes until browned. Repeat with remaining batter.

Nutrition Info: (Per Serving):Calories: 222; Total Fat: 2 g; Saturated Fat: 0 g; Cholesterol: 54 mg; Protein: 9 g; Sodium: 117 mg; Potassium: 541 mg; Fiber: 3 g; Carbohydrates: 42 g; Sugar: 8 g

Sausage And Egg Bake

Servings: 10

Ingredients:

- 1 recipe Peppery Turkey Sausage
- 1 medium onion, chopped
- 1 cup sliced mushrooms
- 1 medium red bell pepper, chopped
- 2 cloves garlic, minced
- 14 large eggs
- 1/2 cup light cream
- 3 tablespoons Mustard
- 1/4 teaspoon pepper

Directions:

1. Preheat oven to 350°F. Spray a 9" × 13" glass baking dish with nonstick cooking spray and set aside.
2. In large skillet, cook sausage, stirring to break up meat, until meat is thoroughly cooked, about 7–8 minutes. Remove sausage from pan and place in baking dish; drain skillet, but do not wipe out.
3. Add onions, mushrooms, bell pepper, and garlic to skillet; cook and stir for 7–9 minutes

or until mushrooms give up their liquid and the liquid evaporates. Place in baking dish on top of sausage.

4. In large bowl, beat eggs with cream, mustard, and pepper until combined. Pour into baking dish on top of sausage and vegetables.

5. Bake for 25–35 minutes or until the eggs are puffy and top just begins to brown. Cut into squares to serve.

Nutrition Info: (Per Serving):Calories: 202; Total Fat: 12 g; Saturated Fat: 3 g; Cholesterol: 331 mg; Protein: 18 g; Sodium: 137 mg; Potassium: 180 mg; Fiber: 0 g; Carbohydrates: 3 g; Sugar: 1 g

Raisin Apple Strata

Servings: 12

Ingredients:

- 3 Granny Smith apples, peeled, cored, and chopped
- 2 tablespoons brown sugar
- 1 tablespoon granulated sugar
- 2 tablespoons orange juice
- 1 teaspoon cinnamon
- 1/4 teaspoon nutmeg
- 16 slices Raisin Bread , cubed
- 1/3 cup maple syrup
- 1/2 cup chopped toasted pecans
- 1/2 cup raisins
- 8 large eggs, beaten
- 13/4 cups whole milk
- 2 teaspoons vanilla

Directions:

1. Preheat oven to 350°F. Spray a 9" × 13" glass baking dish with nonstick cooking spray.
2. Combine chopped apples, brown sugar, granulated sugar, orange juice, cinnamon, and nutmeg in baking dish and toss to coat.

3. Top apples with raisin bread, maple syrup, pecans, and raisins and toss to mix. Spread evenly in baking dish.

4. In large bowl, combine eggs, milk, and vanilla. Pour evenly over bread mixture. Cover and refrigerate overnight.

5. In the morning, uncover the strata. Bake for 55–65 minutes or until the strata is set, with golden brown edges and light golden top. Cut into squares to serve.

Nutrition Info: (Per Serving):Calories: 104; Total Fat: 4 g; Saturated Fat: 1 g; Cholesterol: 38 mg; Protein: 2 g; Sodium: 23 mg; Potassium: 88 mg; Fiber: 1 g; Carbohydrates: 15 g; Sugar: 7 g

Huevos Rancheros

Servings: 4

Ingredients:

- 2 tablespoons (30 ml) vegetable oil
- 4 corn tortillas
- ¼ cup (40 g) onion, chopped
- 2 cups (360 g) tomatoes, chopped
- 2 ounces (55 g) chopped chile peppers
- 4 eggs
- ½ cup (55 g) Swiss cheese, shredded

Directions:

1. In a small skillet, Heat the oil. Cook the tortillas in oil for about 10 seconds on a side, until limp. Line an 8 × 8-inch (20 × 20-cm) baking dish with tortillas. In the same skillet, cook the onion until soft. Stir in the tomatoes and chile peppers. Simmer for about 10 minutes. Spoon over the tortillas. Carefully break the eggs into the skillet. When the whites are set, add a tablespoon of water, cover, and cook until the yolks are almost at desired doneness. Add the eggs over the

sauce in a baking dish. Sprinkle with cheese.
Place under broiler just until cheese melts.

Nutrition Info: (Per Serving): 153 g water; 289 calories (55% from fat, 20% from protein, 25% from carb); 14 g protein; 18 g total fat; 6 g saturated fat; 5 g monounsaturated fat; 5 g polyunsaturated fat; 18 g carb; 3 g fiber; 4 g sugar; 247 mg calcium; 2 mg iron; 102 mg sodium; 375 mg potassium; 1205 IU vitamin A; 44 mg vitamin C; 261 mg cholesterol

Sausage Gravy

Servings: 4

Ingredients:

- ½ pound (225 g) Sausage (see recipe above)
- 3 tablespoons (24 g) all-purpose flour
- 1 cup (235 ml) skim milk
- ¼ teaspoon black pepper

Directions:

1. Remove sausage with a slotted spoon; set aside. Remove all but 2 tablespoons (28 ml) of grease from the skillet. Over medium heat, stir 3 tablespoons (24 g) of flour into the grease. Stir constantly until browned, about 5 minutes. Stirring constantly, pour in milk. Season with pepper. Continue stirring until the gravy is thick. Add sausage back into the gravy. Serve over split biscuits, grits, or mashed potatoes, or pour into a bowl or gravy boat and serve on the side.

Nutrition Info: (Per Serving): 88 g water; 219 calories (64% from fat, 22% from protein, 15% from carb); 12 g protein; 15 g total fat; 5 g saturated fat; 7 g monounsaturated fat; 2 g polyunsaturated fat; 8 g carb; 0 g fiber; 0 g sugar; 95 mg calcium; 1 mg iron; 77 mg sodium; 260 mg potassium; 168 IU vitamin A; 1 mg vitamin C; 42 mg cholesterol

Pear Pecan Muffins

Servings: 18 Muffins

Ingredients:

- 1/2 cup unsalted butter, softened
- 1/4 cup safflower or peanut oil
- 3/4 cup granulated sugar
- 1/2 cup brown sugar
- 2 large eggs
- 2 egg whites
- 1 (15-ounce) can pear halves, drained, reserving liquid
- 1/3 cup lemon juice
- 2 teaspoons vanilla
- 3 cups flour
- 1 teaspoon baking powder
- 1/2 teaspoon baking soda
- 1 cup chopped toasted pecans
- 1 cup powdered sugar

Directions:

1. Preheat oven to 350°F. Line 18 muffin cups with paper liners and set aside, or grease with unsalted butter.

2. In large bowl, combine butter, oil, sugar, and brown sugar and beat until fluffy. Add eggs and egg whites and beat well.

3. Mash the drained pear halves and add to the batter along with lemon juice and vanilla, and mix well.

4. Stir in flour, baking powder, and baking soda and mix just until combined. Stir in pecans.

5. Fill prepared muffin cups 2/3–3/4 full. Bake for 17–22 minutes or until the muffins are light golden brown and spring back when lightly touched. Remove from tins and place on wire racks.

6. In small bowl, combine powdered sugar and 2 tablespoons reserved pear liquid and mix well. Glaze the warm muffins with this mixture, then let cool completely.

Nutrition Info: (Per Serving):Calories: 335; Total Fat: 18 g; Saturated Fat: 4 g; Cholesterol: 37 mg; Protein: 4 g; Sodium: 52 mg; Potassium: 149 mg; Fiber: 2 g; Carbohydrates: 40 g; Sugar: 22 g

Breakfast Mix

Servings: 16

Ingredients:

- 2 cups (200 g) bite-size frosted shredded wheat cereal
- 2 cups (200 g) Kellogg's Cracklin' Oat Bran or other bite-size low sodium cereal
- ½ cup (75 g) dry-roasted peanuts
- ½ cup (82.5 g) raisins
- 2 cups unsalted pretzels
- 3 tablespoons (60 g) honey
- 3 tablespoons (45 ml) corn syrup
- 1 tablespoon (14 g) unsalted butter
- 1 teaspoon ground cinnamon
- ¼ teaspoon ground nutmeg

Directions:

1. Mix cereal, nuts, raisins, and pretzels In a large bowl. Combine the honey, corn syrup, butter, and spices. Microwave until boiling. Pour over cereal mixture, stirring to coat. Place in an ungreased 9 × 13-inch (23 × 33-cm) pan. Bake for 20 minutes at 325°F (170°C, gas mark 3), stirring after 10

minutes. Turn out onto waxed paper. Separate and cool. Store in an airtight container.

Nutrition Info: (Per Serving): 3 g water; 114 calories (24% from fat, 8% from protein, 68% from carb); 3 g protein; 3 g total fat; 1 g saturated fat; 1 g monounsaturated fat; 1 g polyunsaturated fat; 21 g carb; 2 g fiber; 12 g sugar; 12 mg calcium; 5 mg iron; 41 mg sodium; 116 mg potassium; 153 IU vitamin A; 11 mg vitamin C; 2 mg cholesterol

Sausage And Veggie Scrambled Eggs

Servings: 6

Ingredients:

- 1 cup Maple Turkey Sausage
- 2 tablespoons unsalted butter
- 1 medium onion, chopped
- 1/2 cup sliced mushrooms
- 1 medium red bell pepper, chopped
- 6 large eggs, beaten
- 1/4 cup sour cream
- 2 tablespoons milk
- 1/2 teaspoon dried thyme leaves
- 1/8 teaspoon white pepper
- 1/3 cup shredded mozzarella cheese

Directions:

1. In a large skillet over medium heat, cook the sausage, stirring to break up meat, until browned and cooked through. Remove sausage from skillet. Drain fat from skillet, but do not wipe pan.

2. Return skillet to heat and add butter. Add onion, mushrooms, and bell pepper and cook

until vegetables are tender, about 4–5 minutes.

3. Meanwhile, in medium bowl beat eggs, sour cream, milk, thyme, and white pepper until smooth. Pour into skillet over vegetables.

4. Cook, stirring occasionally, and lifting the egg mixture to let uncooked egg flow underneath, until the eggs are just set but still moist.

5. Stir in sausage and add cheese. Cover and let stand off heat 4 minutes, then serve.

Nutrition Info: (Per Serving):Calories: 215; Total Fat: 15 g; Saturated Fat: 7 g; Cholesterol: 248 mg; Protein: 16 g; Sodium: 140 mg; Potassium: 166 mg; Fiber: 0 g; Carbohydrates: 4 g; Sugar: 3 g

Strawberry Egg-white Pancakes

Servings: 4

Ingredients:

- 1/2 cup oats
- 8 egg whites
- 1 tablespoon lemon juice
- 2 tablespoons strawberry jam
- 1/8 cup unbleached all-purpose flour

Directions:

1. Process the oats in a blender or food processor until ground.
2. Whisk the egg whites in a medium metal or glass bowl until soft peaks form.
3. Mix the lemon juice and jam together in a small bowl (this will thin the jam and make it easier to fold into the egg whites).
4. One at a time, fold the thinned jam, ground oatmeal, and flour into the egg whites.
5. Preheat a nonstick pan or griddle treated with cooking spray over medium heat. Pour 1/4 of the mixture into the pan and cook for about 4 minutes or until the top of the pancake bubbles and begins to get dry. Flip

the pancake; cook until the inside of the cake is cooked. Repeat until the remaining 3 pancakes are done.

Nutrition Info: (Per Serving):Calories: 111; Total Fat: 0 g; Saturated Fat: 0 g; Cholesterol: 0 mg; Protein: 9 g; Sodium: 113 mg; Potassium: 160 mg; Fiber: 1 g; Carbohydrates: 17 g; Sugar: 5 g

Lemon Crepes

Servings: 10

Ingredients:

- 2 large eggs
- 3/4 cup unbleached all-purpose flour
- 1 tablespoon lemon juice
- 1/8 teaspoon lemon extract
- 1 cup skim milk
- 1 tablespoon nonfat dry milk
- 1/8 teaspoon baking powder
- Pinch baking soda

Directions:

1. Combine all the ingredients in a blender or food processor and process until the mixture is the consistency of cream.

2. Treat an 8" nonstick skillet with nonstick spray and heat over medium heat. Pour about 2 tablespoons of the crepe batter into the hot pan, tilting in a circular motion until the batter spreads evenly over the pan. Cook the crepe until the outer edges just begin to brown and loosen. Flip the crepe over to the other side and cook for about 30 seconds. Using a thin

spatula, slide the crepe from the pan onto a warm plate or baking sheet set in a warm oven. Continue until all the crepes are done.

3.   Garnish and serve as desired.

Nutrition Info: (Per Serving):Calories: 59; Total Fat: 1 g; Saturated Fat: 0 g; Cholesterol: 42 mg; Protein: 3 g; Sodium: 44 mg; Potassium: 82 mg; Fiber: 0 g; Carbohydrates: 8 g; Sugar: 1 g

Cinnamon Rolls

Servings: 9

Ingredients:

- For dough:
- 1 cup (235 ml) water
- 2 tablespoons (28 ml) vegetable oil
- 1 egg
- 3 cups (330 g) bread flour
- ¼ cup (50 g) sugar
- 3 teaspoons (12 g) yeast
- For filling:
- ⅓ cup (67 g) sugar
- 2 teaspoons (5 g) ground cinnamon
- 2 tablespoons (28 g) unsalted butter, softened

Directions:

1. Place dough ingredients in bread machine in the order specified by manufacturer. Process on dough cycle. Remove dough and press out to a 9 × 18-inch (23 × 46-cm) rectangle on a lightly floured board. Mix together cinnamon and sugar. Spread dough with softened butter, then sprinkle with cinnamon-sugar mixture.

Roll up tightly, beginning on the 9-inch (23-cm) side. Slice into 9 slices. Place cut side down in a greased 9 × 9-inch (23 × 23-cm) baking pan. Cover and let rise until doubled, 30 to 45 minutes. Bake at 375°F (190°C, gas mark 5) until golden, 25 to 30 minutes.

Nutrition Info: (Per Serving): 38 g water; 280 calories (23% from fat, 10% from protein, 67% from carb); 7 g protein; 7 g total fat; 2 g saturated fat; 2 g monounsaturated fat; 2 g polyunsaturated fat; 47 g carb; 2 g fiber; 13 g sugar; 19 mg calcium; 3 mg iron; 12 mg sodium; 85 mg potassium; 112 IU vitamin A; 0 mg vitamin C; 34 mg cholesterol

Banana Walnut Breakfast Cookies

Servings: 24 Cookies

Ingredients:

- 1/3 cup unsalted butter, softened
- 1/3 cup unsalted peanut butter
- 2 medium bananas, mashed
- 1 large egg
- 1/2 cup brown sugar
- 2 tablespoons honey
- 2 teaspoons vanilla
- 1 cup all-purpose flour
- 1/4 cup whole-wheat flour
- 1/2 teaspoon baking powder
- 11/2 cups rolled oats
- 1 cup dried cherries
- 1/2 cup chopped walnuts

Directions:

1. Preheat oven to 350°F.
2. In large bowl, combine butter and peanut butter and mix well. Add mashed banana and egg and stir until combined.
3. Beat in brown sugar, honey, and vanilla and mix well. Add flour, whole-wheat flour, baking

powder, and oats and mix until combined. Stir in cherries and walnuts.

4.   Drop dough by tablespoons onto a cookie sheet. Bake for 11–16 minutes or until the cookies are light golden brown and set. Remove to wire rack to cool completely before storing.

Nutrition Info: (Per Serving):Calories: 141; Total Fat: 6 g; Saturated Fat: 2 g; Cholesterol: 15 mg; Protein: 3 g; Sodium: 5 mg; Potassium: 123 mg; Fiber: 1 g; Carbohydrates: 18 g; Sugar: 8 g

Farro Porridge With Nuts

Servings: 4

Ingredients:

- 1 cup farro, rinsed
- 3/4 cup water
- 3/4 cup almond milk
- 1/3 cup orange juice
- 1/4 cup brown sugar
- 1 teaspoon vanilla
- 1/3 cup chopped walnuts, toasted
- 1/3 cup chopped cashews, toasted

Directions:

1. Combine the farro, water, almond milk, orange juice, and brown sugar in a medium saucepan over medium heat. Bring to a boil, stirring occasionally.
2. Reduce heat to low and cook, stirring occasionally, until the mixture is creamy and the farro is tender but still chewy, about 25 minutes. Stir in vanilla and nuts and serve immediately.

Nutrition Info: (Per Serving):Calories: 402; Total Fat: 14 g; Saturated Fat: 1 g; Cholesterol: 0 mg; Protein:

11 g; Sodium: 32 mg; Potassium: 186 mg; Fiber: 8 g; Carbohydrates: 57 g; Sugar: 16 g

Pancakes

Servings: 3

Ingredients:

- 1 ¼ cups (145 g) all-purpose flour
- 2 tablespoons (26 g) sugar
- 2 teaspoons (9 g) sodium-free baking powder
- 1 egg
- 1 cup (235 ml) milk
- 1 tablespoon (15 ml) vegetable oil

Directions:

1. In a mixing bowl, stir together the dry ingredients. Combine the egg, milk, and oil. Add all at once to the flour mixture. Stir until blended but still slightly lumpy. Pour about ¼ cup of batter onto hot greased griddle for each pancake. Cook until browned on bottom (when bubbles form and then break). Turn and cook on other side until done.

Nutrition Info: (Per Serving): 95 g water; 322 calories (20% from fat, 13% from protein, 67% from carb); 11 g protein; 7 g total fat; 1 g saturated fat; 2 g monounsaturated fat; 3 g polyunsaturated fat; 54 g

carb; 1 g fiber; 13 g sugar; 265 mg calcium; 3 mg iron; 65 mg sodium; 546 mg potassium; 261 IU vitamin A; 0 mg vitamin C; 83 mg cholesterol

Sausage

Servings: 8

Ingredients:

- 1 pound (455 g) pork, ground
- ¼ teaspoon black pepper
- ¼ teaspoon white pepper
- ¾ teaspoon dried sage
- ¼ teaspoon mace
- ½ teaspoon garlic powder
- ¼ teaspoon onion powder
- ¼ teaspoon ground allspice

Directions:

1. Combine all ingredients, mixing well. Fry, grill, or cook on a greased baking sheet in a 325°F (170°C, gas mark 3) oven until done.

Nutrition Info: (Per Serving): 38 g water; 121 calories (60% from fat, 38% from protein, 1% from carb); 11 g protein; 8 g total fat; 3 g saturated fat; 4 g monounsaturated fat; 1 g polyunsaturated fat; 0 g carb; 0 g fiber; 0 g sugar; 5 mg calcium; 0 mg iron; 24 mg sodium; 223 mg potassium; 8 IU vitamin A; 0 mg vitamin C; 34 mg cholesterol

Apple Pancakes

Servings: 6

Ingredients:

- 1 ½ cups (165 g) all-purpose flour
- 2 tablespoons (26 g) sugar
- 1 tablespoon (14 g) sodium-free baking powder
- ¼ teaspoon ground nutmeg
- 2 eggs
- 1 cup (235 ml) skim milk
- 1 cup (245 g) applesauce
- 2 tablespoons (28 g) unsalted butter, melted

Directions:

1. Combine dry ingredients In a large mixing bowl. Beat together eggs, milk, applesauce, and butter. Add to dry ingredients and stir until just mixed, but still lumpy. Heat griddle and pour about 1/4 cup (60 ml) for each pancake. Allow to cook until bubbles burst. Flip and cook until golden.

Nutrition Info: (Per Serving): 90 g water; 244 calories (23% from fat, 12% from protein, 65% from carb); 7 g protein; 6 g total fat; 1 g saturated fat; 3 g monounsaturated fat; 2 g polyunsaturated fat; 40 g carb; 1 g fiber; 4 g sugar; 185 mg calcium; 2 mg iron; 66 mg sodium; 414 mg potassium; 350 IU vitamin A; 1 mg vitamin C; 83 mg cholesterol

Almond-butter Cranberry Oatmeal Bars

Servings: 36

Ingredients:

- 1/3 cup no-salt-added almond butter
- 2/3 cup unsalted butter, melted
- 1/2 cup granulated sugar
- 1/2 cup brown sugar
- 1/4 cup honey
- 2 teaspoons vanilla
- 3 cups rolled oats
- 2/3 cup dried cranberries
- 1/2 cup slivered almonds

Directions:

1. Preheat oven to 375°F. Spray a 13" × 9" pan with nonstick baking spray containing flour and set aside.
2. In large bowl, combine almond butter, butter, granulated sugar, brown sugar, and honey and mix well.
3. Beat in vanilla, then stir in oats, cranberries, and almonds. Press into prepared pan.

4. Bake for 15–20 minutes or until the edges are golden brown and mixture is set. Let cool completely, then cut into bars.

Nutrition Info: (Per Serving):Calories: 114; Total Fat: 6 g; Saturated Fat: 2 g; Cholesterol: 8 mg; Protein: 1 g; Sodium: 2 mg; Potassium: 61 mg; Fiber: 1 g; Carbohydrates: 14 g; Sugar: 9 g

Apple Turnovers

Servings: 9

Ingredients:

- 3 Granny Smith or Braeburn apples, peeled, cored, and chopped
- 2 tablespoons unsalted butter
- 2/3 cup brown sugar
- 1 teaspoon cinnamon
- 1/4 teaspoon nutmeg
- 1 tablespoon flour
- 1 tablespoon orange juice
- 2 teaspoons vanilla, divided
- 1/3 cup dried cherries, chopped
- 1/3 cup chopped toasted pecans
- 1 (17-ounce) package frozen puff pastry, thawed
- 11/4 cups powdered sugar
- 1–2 tablespoons cherry juice

Directions:

1. In medium saucepan over medium heat, combine chopped apples, butter, brown sugar, cinnamon, and nutmeg. Cook, stirring, until apples are tender, about 5 minutes.

2. In small bowl, combine flour and orange juice and mix well. Stir into apple mixture and cook, stirring, for another 1–2 minutes or until mixture has thickened.

3. Remove apple mixture from heat, stir in 1 teaspoon vanilla, dried cherries, and pecans, and set aside to cool for 45 minutes.

4. When apple mixture has cooled for 45 minutes, preheat oven to 400°F.

5. Unfold the puff pastry sheets and place on lightly floured board. Cut each sheet into 4 squares, making 8 squares total.

6. Divide the apple mixture among the squares. Fold the puff pastry over the apples to make triangles. Press edges with a fork to seal.

7. Place turnovers on a parchment paper–lined baking sheet. Bake for 20–30 minutes or until turnovers are puffed and light golden brown. Cool on wire rack.

8. To make the glaze: combine powdered sugar, cherry juice, and 1 teaspoon vanilla in a medium bowl until a thick glaze forms. Drizzle this over the cooled turnovers and let stand until set.

Nutrition Info: (Per Serving):Calories: 541; Total Fat: 30 g; Saturated Fat: 7 g; Cholesterol: 6 mg; Protein: 5 g; Sodium: 139 mg; Potassium: 162 mg; Fiber: 3 g; Carbohydrates: 64 g; Sugar: 37 g

Soft Granola Bars

Servings: 27

Ingredients:

- 3 cups (240 g) quick-cooking oats
- ½ cup (115 g) brown sugar
- ¼ cup (28 g) wheat germ
- ½ cup (112 g) unsalted butter
- ¼ cup (60 ml) corn syrup
- ¼ cup (85 g) honey
- ½ cup (82.5 g) raisins
- ½ cup (35 g) sweetened coconut

Directions:

1. Combine the oats, sugar, and wheat germ. Cut in the butter until the mixture is crumbly. Stir in the corn syrup and honey. Add the raisins and coconut. Press into a greased 9-inch (23-cm) square pan. Bake at 350°F (180°C, gas mark 4) for 20 to 25 minutes. Let cool for 10 minutes, then cut into bars.

Nutrition Info: (Per Serving): 4 g water; 153 calories (30% from fat, 8% from protein, 61% from carb); 3 g protein; 5 g total fat; 3 g saturated fat; 1 g monounsaturated fat; 1 g polyunsaturated fat; 24 g

carb; 2 g fiber; 11 g sugar; 16 mg calcium; 1 mg iron; 11 mg sodium; 129 mg potassium; 105 IU vitamin A; 0 mg vitamin C; 9 mg cholesterol

Wild Rice Waffles

Servings: 4

Ingredients:

- 2/3 cup wild rice
- 11/3 cups water
- 11/3 cups flour
- 1 tablespoon cornstarch
- 1/2 teaspoon baking powder
- 1/2 teaspoon cinnamon, if desired
- 3 large eggs
- 2 tablespoons sugar
- 3/4 cup milk
- 2 tablespoons orange juice
- 1/4 cup unsalted butter, melted

Directions:

1. In small saucepan, combine wild rice and water. Bring to a boil over high heat, then reduce heat to low, cover, and simmer for 35–45 minutes or until rice is just tender. Drain, if necessary, and spread on a plate to cool.

2. When rice is cool, combine flour, cornstarch, and baking powder (and cinnamon, if using) in a medium bowl and mix.

3. In a large bowl, beat eggs with sugar until light and lemon colored. Beat in milk, orange juice, and melted butter. Fold in flour mixture. Fold in wild rice.

4. Preheat your waffle iron. Make waffles according to manufacturer's instructions. Serve immediately with maple syrup and fresh berries.

Nutrition Info: (Per Serving):Calories: 460; Total Fat: 16 g; Saturated Fat: 9 g; Cholesterol: 192 mg; Protein: 14 g; Sodium: 77 mg; Potassium: 356 mg; Fiber: 3 g; Carbohydrates: 63 g; Sugar: 10 g

Veggie Frittata

Servings: 4

Ingredients:

- 1 cup grape tomatoes, chopped
- 1 tablespoon sliced fresh basil leaves
- 1 tablespoon minced green onion
- 2 tablespoons olive oil
- 1/2 cup diced red onion
- 1/2 cup chopped red bell pepper
- 1/2 cup chopped peeled zucchini
- 1/2 cup chopped mushrooms
- 6 large eggs
- 1/3 cup whole milk
- 1/2 teaspoon dried basil leaves
- 1/8 teaspoon white pepper
- 2 tablespoons grated Parmesan cheese

Directions:

1. Use an ovenproof 8" skillet, or cover the wooden handle of a skillet with foil to protect it.
2. In small bowl, combine grape tomatoes, fresh basil, and green onion and set aside.

3. In the skillet, heat olive oil over medium heat. Add red onion, bell pepper, zucchini, and mushrooms and cook until lightly browned, about 6–7 minutes.

4. Meanwhile, in medium bowl combine eggs, milk, dried basil, and white pepper, and beat well. Pour into skillet over vegetables.

5. Cook over medium heat for 5–10 minutes, lifting egg mixture occasionally to let uncooked egg flow underneath and shaking pan, until the bottom is golden brown.

6. Meanwhile, preheat broiler to high. Sprinkle frittata with cheese and place under broiler. Broil for 10–12 minutes, moving skillet around under the broiler, until frittata is set and top is light golden brown.

7. Cut frittata into wedges and serve with the grape-tomato mixture for a topping.

Nutrition Info: (Per Serving):Calories: 223; Total Fat: 16 g; Saturated Fat: 4 g; Cholesterol: 320 mg; Protein: 12 g; Sodium: 137 mg; Potassium: 397 mg; Fiber: 1 g; Carbohydrates: 8 g; Sugar: 6 g

Apple Strata

Servings: 4

Ingredients:

- 3 cups low sodium bread, cubed
- 1 can (15 ounces, or 455 g) apples
- 3 ounces (85 g) Swiss cheese, shredded
- 4 eggs
- ¼ cup (60 ml) skim milk

Directions:

1. Cube bread and place in a 9-inch-square (23-cm-square) pan sprayed with nonstick vegetable oil spray. Spoon apples over bread. Sprinkle with cheese. Combine eggs and milk and pour over bread, apples, and cheese. Cover with plastic wrap and refrigerate overnight. Heat oven to 350°F (180°C, gas mark 4). Bake uncovered for 40 to 45 minutes or until top is lightly browned and center is set.

Nutrition Info: (Per Serving): 106 g water; 277 calories (42% from fat, 24% from protein, 33% from carb); 17 g protein; 13 g total fat; 6 g saturated fat; 4 g monounsaturated fat; 1 g polyunsaturated fat; 23 g

carb; 1 g fiber; 5 g sugar; 295 mg calcium; 2 mg iron; 102 mg sodium; 198 mg potassium; 500 IU vitamin A; 1 mg vitamin C; 266 mg cholesterol

Kedgeree

Servings: 4

Ingredients:

- 1 cup basmati rice
- 2 teaspoons curry powder
- 1/2 teaspoon turmeric
- 2 cups chicken stock
- 2 (6-ounce) salmon fillets
- 4 large eggs
- 1/4 cup light cream
- 1/8 teaspoon white pepper
- 2 tablespoons unsalted butter
- 2 tablespoons lemon juice
- 1/4 cup chopped flat-leaf parsley

Directions:

1. In medium saucepan, combine rice, curry powder, and turmeric. Add chicken stock and bring to a simmer over high heat. Reduce heat to low, cover, and cook for 15–20 minutes or until rice is tender and liquid is absorbed. Remove from heat.

2. Place salmon on a broiler pan. Broil 6" from heat for 8–9 minutes until salmon is just

cooked through and flakes when tested with a fork. Set aside.

3.   In small bowl, beat eggs with cream and pepper.

4.   Melt butter in a medium skillet over medium heat. Add the eggs to the saucepan and cook them, stirring, until curds form. When eggs are just cooked, but still soft and shiny, remove from heat.

5.   Fluff the rice with a fork. Stir in the salmon, eggs, lemon juice, and parsley. Serve immediately.

Nutrition Info: (Per Serving):Calories: 491; Total Fat: 22 g; Saturated Fat: 8 g; Cholesterol: 290 mg; Protein: 30 g; Sodium: 132 mg; Potassium: 625 mg; Fiber: 1 g; Carbohydrates: 41 g; Sugar: 1 g

Cinnamon Pull-apart Loaf

Servings: 12

Ingredients:

- 4 tablespoons (60 g) sugar, divided
- 1 ½ teaspoons ground cinnamon
- 3 ½ cups (385 g) Buttermilk Baking Mix
- ⅔ cup (157 ml) skim milk
- 2 tablespoons (28 g) unsalted butter
- 1 teaspoon vanilla extract
- 1 egg
- ½ cup (50 g) powdered sugar
- 2 tablespoons (30 ml) water

Directions:

1. Mix 2 tablespoons sugar and the cinnamon. Place in a resealable plastic bag. Spray a 9 × 5 × 3-inch (23 × 13 × 7.5-cm) loaf pan with nonstick vegetable oil spray. Stir together the baking mix, milk, remaining sugar, butter, vanilla, and egg until it forms a ball. Pinch off 1 ½-inch (4-cm) pieces. Shake in the cinnamon-sugar mixture until coated and then place in the pan. Bake at 375°F (190°C, gas mark 5) for 25 to 30 minutes or until golden

brown. Let stand in pan for 10 minutes before removing. Mix together powdered sugar and water and drizzle over top.

Nutrition Info: (Per Serving): 22 g water; 209 calories (33% from fat, 7% from protein, 60% from carb); 4 g protein; 8 g total fat; 3 g saturated fat; 4 g monounsaturated fat; 1 g polyunsaturated fat; 31 g carb; 1 g fiber; 13 g sugar; 86 mg calcium; 1 mg iron; 21 mg sodium; 88 mg potassium; 113 IU vitamin A; 0 mg vitamin C; 26 mg cholesterol

Spiced Apple Egg Clouds On Toast

Servings: 2

Ingredients:

- 4 egg whites
- 1 teaspoon powdered sugar, sifted
- 2 teaspoons unsalted butter
- 1 large apple, peeled, cored, and thinly sliced
- 2 teaspoons lemon juice
- 1 teaspoon brown sugar
- 1/4 teaspoon cinnamon
- Pinch ground cloves
- Pinch ground ginger
- Pinch ground allspice
- 2 cups water
- 2 slices low-salt bread
- Optional: Freshly ground nutmeg

Directions:

1. In a medium metal or glass bowl, beat the egg whites until they thicken. Add the powdered sugar, and continue to beat until stiff peaks form.

2. Heat a small sauté pan over medium heat; add the butter. Toss the apple slices in the lemon juice and add them to the pan. Sprinkle the brown sugar, cinnamon, cloves, ginger, and allspice over the apples; sauté, stirring occasionally, until the apples are tender and glazed, about 5–6 minutes.

3. While the apples cook, bring the water to a simmer in a large, deep nonstick sauté pan over medium-low heat. Drop the egg whites by the tablespoonful into the simmering water. Simmer for 3 minutes, then turn the egg white "clouds" over, and simmer for an additional 3 minutes. Remove egg white clouds from pan with a large strainer one at a time, and briefly drain on paper towels to remove excess water.

4. Toast the bread and divide the apples over the slices, then top with the "clouds." Sprinkle with nutmeg, if desired. Serve immediately.

Nutrition Info: (Per Serving):Calories: 190; Total Fat: 4 g; Saturated Fat: 2 g; Cholesterol: 10 mg; Protein: 9 g; Sodium: 116 mg; Potassium: 242 mg; Fiber: 2 g; Carbohydrates: 28 g; Sugar: 13 g

Hard-cooked Eggs

Servings: 8

Ingredients:

- 8 large eggs

Directions:

1. Place the eggs in a large saucepan and add cold water to cover. Bring to a boil over high heat.
2. When the water comes to a rolling boil, cover the pan, remove it from heat, and let stand for 15 minutes.
3. Then place the pan with the eggs in the sink. Run cold water into the pan until the eggs are cold.
4. Crack the eggs under the water and let sit for 5 minutes; then peel.
5. Or put one egg into a glass and add a little water. Cover the top with your hand and shake well over the sink. The shell should slip right off.
6. Cover the eggs and store in the fridge up to 4 days.

Nutrition Info: (Per Serving):Calories: 77; Total Fat: 5 g; Saturated Fat: 1 g; Cholesterol: 212 mg; Protein: 6 g; Sodium: 62 mg; Potassium: 63 mg; Fiber: 0 g; Carbohydrates: 0 g; Sugar: 0 g

Power Bars

Servings: 12

Ingredients:

- 1 cup (80 g) quick-cooking oats
- ½ cup (75 g) whole wheat flour
- ½ cup (57 g) Grape-Nuts cereal, or other nugget-type cereal
- ½ teaspoon ground cinnamon
- 1 egg
- ¼ cup (60 g) applesauce
- ¼ cup (85 g) honey
- 3 tablespoons (45 g) brown sugar
- 2 tablespoons (30 ml) vegetable oil
- ¼ cup (56 g) sunflower seeds, unsalted
- ¼ cup (35 g) walnuts, chopped
- 7 ounces (198 g) dried fruit

Directions:

1. Preheat oven to 325°F (170°C, gas mark 3). Line a 9-inch (23-cm) square baking pan with aluminum foil. Spray the foil with cooking spray. In a large bowl, stir together the oats, flour, cereal, and cinnamon. Add the egg, applesauce, honey, brown sugar, and oil. Mix

well. Stir in the sunflower seeds, walnuts, and dried fruit. Spread mixture evenly in the prepared pan. Bake for 30 minutes, or until firm and lightly browned around the edges. Let cool. Use the foil to lift from the pan. Cut into bars and store in the refrigerator.

Nutrition Info: (Per Serving): 16 g water; 223 calories (26% from fat, 10% from protein, 65% from carb); 6 g protein; 7 g total fat; 1 g saturated fat; 2 g monounsaturated fat; 4 g polyunsaturated fat; 38 g carb; 4 g fiber; 10 g sugar; 27 mg calcium; 3 mg iron; 43 mg sodium; 285 mg potassium; 493 IU vitamin A; 1 mg vitamin C; 20 mg cholesterol

Honey-topped Coffee Cake

Servings: 8

Ingredients:

- 1 ½ cups (165 g) all-purpose flour
- ½ cup (100 g) sugar
- 2 teaspoons (9 g) sodium-free baking powder
- ½ teaspoon mace
- 1 can (8 ¾ ounces, or 255 g) pineapple, crushed
- 1 egg
- ¼ cup (60 ml) vegetable oil
- ⅓ cup (115 g) honey
- ½ cup (57 g) granola
- ¼ cup (18 g) coconut

Directions:

1. Stir together dry ingredients. Drain pineapple, reserving syrup. Add water to syrup if necessary to make ½ cup. Combine syrup, egg, and oil. Add to flour mixture, stirring until smooth. Pour into 9 × 1 ½-inch (23 × 4-cm) round baking pan sprayed with nonstick vegetable oil spray. Combine honey,

68

pineapple, granola, and coconut. Spread over batter. Bake at 400°F (200°C, gas mark 6) until done, about 25 minutes.

Nutrition Info: (Per Serving): 38 g water; 314 calories (29% from fat, 6% from protein, 65% from carb); 5 g protein; 10 g total fat; 2 g saturated fat; 3 g monounsaturated fat; 5 g polyunsaturated fat; 52 g carb; 2 g fiber; 30 g sugar; 73 mg calcium; 2 mg iron; 15 mg sodium; 250 mg potassium; 49 IU vitamin A; 3 mg vitamin C; 31 mg cholesterol

Fruit Smoothie

Servings: 2

Ingredients:

- 1/2 cup frozen strawberries, unsweetened
- 1 tablespoon apple juice concentrate
- 3 tablespoons water
- 1/2 medium banana, sliced
- 8 ounces peach nonfat yogurt

Directions:

1. Put all the ingredients in a blender or food processor and process until thick and smooth. Serve immediately.

Nutrition Info: (Per Serving):Calories: 158; Total Fat: 0 g; Saturated Fat: 0 g; Cholesterol: 2 mg; Protein: 5 g; Sodium: 68 mg; Potassium: 411 mg; Fiber: 1 g; Carbohydrates: 34 g; Sugar: 29 g

Baked Savory Oatmeal

Servings: 4

Ingredients:

- 2 tablespoons unsalted butter, plus more for greasing
- 1 medium red onion, chopped
- 1 clove garlic, minced
- 1 cup sliced mushrooms
- 11/4 cups rolled oats (not instant or quick cooking)
- 11/4 cups whole milk
- 1 large egg, beaten
- 1/2 teaspoon dried thyme leaves
- 2 tablespoons grated Parmesan cheese

Directions:

1. Preheat oven to 375°F. Grease a 9" square pan with unsalted butter and set aside.
2. In medium skillet, melt butter over medium heat. Add onion, garlic, and mushrooms and cook until tender, stirring occasionally, about 4–5 minutes. Remove from heat and place in medium bowl.

3. Add oats, milk, egg, and thyme to mixture in bowl and mix well. Spoon into prepared pan. Sprinkle with cheese.

4. Bake for 30–40 minutes or until top is light golden brown and the mixture is set. Cut into squares to serve with maple syrup, if desired.

Nutrition Info: (Per Serving):Calories: 253; Total Fat: 11 g; Saturated Fat: 6 g; Cholesterol: 78 mg; Protein: 9 g; Sodium: 96 mg; Potassium: 381 mg; Fiber: 3 g; Carbohydrates: 27 g; Sugar: 8 g

Peppery Turkey Sausage

Servings: 8

Ingredients:

- 1 pound lean ground turkey
- 1/4 teaspoon garlic powder
- 1/4 teaspoon onion powder
- 1/4 teaspoon dried sage
- 1/2 teaspoon freshly ground black pepper
- 1/8 teaspoon ground cloves
- Pinch ground allspice

Directions:

1. In a mixing bowl, combine all the ingredients until well mixed. Form into 8 equal-sized patties.

2. Pan-fry on a nonstick grill pan or prepare in a covered indoor grill (such as a George Foreman–style indoor grill). The sausage is done when the juices run clear and a food thermometer registers 165°F. You can also cook the sausage as you would any ground meat, stirring to break up the meat.

Nutrition Info: (Per Serving):Calories: 76; Total Fat: 3 g; Saturated Fat: 0 g; Cholesterol: 32 mg; Protein: 11

g; Sodium: 40 mg; Potassium: 4 mg; Fiber: 0 g; Carbohydrates: 0 g; Sugar: 0 g

Baked Cranberry Orange Oatmeal With Orange Sauce

Servings: 8

Ingredients:

- 21/2 cups rolled oats
- 1/2 cup chopped pecans
- 1/2 cup brown sugar
- 1/2 teaspoon cinnamon
- 1/8 teaspoon cardamom
- 1 teaspoon grated orange rind
- 2/3 cup dried cranberries
- 1 cup whole milk
- 1 cup light cream
- 11/3 cups orange juice, divided
- 2 large eggs
- 1/4 cup unsalted butter, melted, divided
- 1 tablespoon cornstarch
- 1/4 cup granulated sugar
- 1 tablespoon unsalted butter

Directions:

1. Preheat oven to 375°F. Grease a 13" × 9" pan with unsalted butter and set aside.

2. In large bowl, combine oats, pecans, brown sugar, cinnamon, cardamom, orange rind, and cranberries, and mix well.

3. In medium bowl, combine milk, cream, 1/3 cup orange juice, eggs, and half of the melted butter and beat well.

4. Stir the milk mixture into the oats. Spread into prepared pan and drizzle with remaining melted butter.

5. Bake for 35–45 minutes or until top is golden and the mixture is set.

6. Meanwhile, combine 1 cup orange juice, cornstarch, granulated sugar, and 1 tablespoon unsalted butter in a small saucepan and bring to a boil. Reduce heat to low and simmer for 3–4 minutes until thickened.

7. Slice the baked oatmeal into squares and serve drizzled with the orange sauce.

Nutrition Info: (Per Serving):Calories: 430; Total Fat: 21 g; Saturated Fat: 9 g; Cholesterol: 94 mg; Protein: 7 g; Sodium: 48 mg; Potassium: 324 mg; Fiber: 4 g; Carbohydrates: 53 g; Sugar: 31 g

Dutch Baby

Servings: 4

Ingredients:

- 2 tablespoons sugar
- 3 large eggs, at room temperature
- 11/2 teaspoons vanilla
- 1/2 cup whole milk
- 2 tablespoons lemon juice
- 1/2 cup plus 2 tablespoons flour
- 1 tablespoon cornstarch
- 1/8 teaspoon cinnamon
- 1/4 cup unsalted butter
- 2 tablespoons powdered sugar
- 1 cup fresh raspberries
- 1/2 cup chopped strawberries
- 1 tablespoon chopped fresh mint
- 1/3 cup maple syrup

Directions:

1. Preheat oven to 425°F. Place a 10" ovenproof skillet in the oven to heat.
2. In large bowl, combine sugar with eggs and vanilla and beat until light and fluffy. Beat in milk and lemon juice.

3. In small bowl, combine flour, cornstarch, and cinnamon and mix well. Beat into egg mixture until smooth.

4. Carefully, using a pot holder, remove the hot skillet from the oven and let sit for 2 minutes. Add butter to skillet and swirl to coat the bottom and sides.

5. Pour the batter into the skillet; it will start sizzling. Immediately place into the oven. Bake for 16–20 minutes or until puffed and light golden.

6. Remove the skillet from the oven; the pancake will sink. Sprinkle with powdered sugar, then fill with the berries and mint and serve with maple syrup.

Nutrition Info: (Per Serving):Calories: 392; Total Fat: 16 g; Saturated Fat: 9 g; Cholesterol: 192 mg; Protein: 8 g; Sodium: 70 mg; Potassium: 266 mg; Fiber: 3 g; Carbohydrates: 52 g; Sugar: 30 g

Streusel French Toast

Servings: 8

Ingredients:

- 8 (1") slices French Bread or other bread , cut on the diagonal
- 3 large eggs
- 1 cup whole milk
- 1/4 cup plus 3 tablespoons granulated sugar, divided
- 1/2 cup plus 2 tablespoons unsalted butter, melted, divided
- 11/2 teaspoons cinnamon, divided
- 1/8 teaspoon cardamom
- 1 teaspoon vanilla
- 1/2 cup brown sugar
- 1/2 cup flour
- 1/2 cup rolled oats
- 1/2 cup chopped pecans

Directions:

1. Place the bread slices in a greased 9" × 13" glass baking dish.
2. In medium bowl, combine eggs, milk, 1/4 cup granulated sugar, 2 tablespoons melted

butter, 1/2 teaspoon cinnamon, cardamom, and vanilla and mix well. Pour over the French bread, saturating each piece. Cover with foil and refrigerate overnight.

3.   In small bowl, combine brown sugar, flour, oats, pecans, 3 tablespoons granulated sugar, and 1 teaspoon cinnamon and mix. Add 1/2 cup melted butter and mix until crumbly. Cover with foil and refrigerate overnight.

4.   In the morning, preheat oven to 375°F. Uncover the pan with the bread. Sprinkle each piece of bread with some of the oat-streusel mixture.

5.   Bake for 30–40 minutes or until the bread is golden brown. Serve immediately with maple syrup.

Nutrition Info: (Per Serving):Calories: 475; Total Fat: 28 g; Saturated Fat: 11 g; Cholesterol: 119 mg; Protein: 8 g; Sodium: 68 mg; Potassium: 204 mg; Fiber: 3 g; Carbohydrates: 48 g; Sugar: 22 g

Oven Omelet

Servings: 6

Ingredients:

- 2 tablespoons unsalted butter, divided
- 1/3 cup chopped mushrooms
- 1/4 cup chopped yellow summer squash
- 2 tablespoons chopped green onions
- 6 large eggs
- 1/2 cup milk
- 1/2 teaspoon dried thyme leaves
- 1/8 teaspoon pepper
- 1/2 cup shredded whole milk mozzarella cheese

Directions:

1. Preheat oven to 375°F. Grease a 9" glass pie plate with 1 teaspoon unsalted butter and set aside.

2. In small skillet over medium heat, melt remaining butter. Add mushrooms, squash, and green onions; cook and stir for 4–5 minutes or until vegetables are tender. Arrange in prepared pie plate.

3. In medium bowl, combine eggs, milk, thyme, and pepper and beat well. Pour over vegetables in pie plate. Sprinkle with cheese.

4. Bake for 20–30 minutes or until set. Cut into wedges to serve.

Nutrition Info: (Per Serving):Calories: 146; Total Fat: 11 g; Saturated Fat: 5 g; Cholesterol: 231 mg; Protein: 9 g; Sodium: 138 mg; Potassium: 138 mg; Fiber: 0 g; Carbohydrates: 2 g; Sugar: 1 g

Glazed Lemon Muffins

Servings: 12 Muffins

Ingredients:

- 11/2 cups flour
- 1/3 cup almond flour
- 3 tablespoons ground coconut
- 1 teaspoon baking powder
- 1/2 teaspoon baking soda
- 1 cup granulated sugar
- 1/2 cup milk
- 1/3 cup sour cream
- 4 tablespoons lemon juice, divided
- 1 teaspoon grated lemon zest, divided
- 1 teaspoon vanilla
- 1/4 cup unsalted butter, melted
- 1 large egg
- 11/2 cups powdered sugar

Directions:

1. Preheat oven to 375°F. Line a 12-cup muffin tin with paper liners and set aside, or spray each cup with nonstick baking spray containing flour.

2. In large bowl, combine flour, almond flour, ground coconut, baking powder, baking soda, and granulated sugar and whisk to combine.

3. In small bowl, combine milk, sour cream, 2 tablespoons lemon juice, 1/2 teaspoon lemon zest, vanilla, melted butter, and egg and beat until smooth.

4. Stir milk mixture into dry ingredients and stir just until combined.

5. Spoon batter into prepared muffin tins. Bake for 17–22 minutes or until the muffins are very light golden brown and spring back when lightly touched with your finger.

6. While muffins are baking, combine powdered sugar, 2 tablespoons lemon juice, and 1/2 teaspoon zest in small bowl. When the muffins are done baking (and still in the pan), drizzle some of this glaze over each muffin, using about half of the glaze.

7. Remove muffins from muffin tin and let cool on wire rack. When cool, drizzle with remaining glaze.

Nutrition Info: (Per Serving):Calories: 257; Total Fat: 8 g; Saturated Fat: 4 g; Cholesterol: 28 mg; Protein: 3

g; Sodium: 72 mg; Potassium: 105 mg; Fiber: 1 g; Carbohydrates: 43 g; Sugar: 30 g

Banana Fritters

Servings: 4

Ingredients:

- 1 cup (110 g) all-purpose flour
- 1 tablespoon (15 g) sugar
- 1 tablespoon (14 g) sodium-free baking powder
- ½ cup (120 ml) skim milk
- 1 egg
- 1 tablespoon (15 ml) canola oil
- 1 cup (225 g) banana, chopped
- ½ teaspoon ground nutmeg

Directions:

1. Stir together flour, sugar, and baking powder. Combine the milk, egg, and oil. Add banana and nutmeg. Stir into dry ingredients, stirring until just moistened. Drop by tablespoonfuls into hot oil. Fry for 2 to 3 minutes on a side until golden brown. Drain.

Nutrition Info: (Per Serving): 85 g water; 245 calories (20% from fat, 11% from protein, 69% from carb); 7 g protein; 6 g total fat; 1 g saturated fat; 3 g monounsaturated fat; 1 g polyunsaturated fat; 44 g

carb; 2 g fiber; 10 g sugar; 222 mg calcium; 2 mg iron; 43 mg sodium; 690 mg potassium; 169 IU vitamin A; 5 mg vitamin C; 62 mg cholesterol

Chicken Salad On Wild Rice Waffles

Servings: 4

Ingredients:

- 4 Wild Rice Waffles , toasted
- 4 cups Chicken Wild Rice Salad

Directions:

1. While waffles are still hot, top each with a cup of the chicken salad. Serve immediately.

Nutrition Info: (Per Serving):Calories: 584; Total Fat: 25 g; Saturated Fat: 4 g; Cholesterol: 71 mg; Protein: 35 g; Sodium: 95 mg; Potassium: 664 mg; Fiber: 4 g; Carbohydrates: 56 g; Sugar: 14 g

Overnight Fruit And Oatmeal

Servings: 4

Ingredients:

- 1 cup steel-cut oats
- 14 dried apricot halves, chopped
- 1 dried fig, chopped
- 2 tablespoons golden raisins
- 4 cups water
- 1/2 cup whole milk
- 1/4 teaspoon cinnamon
- 1/8 teaspoon grated orange zest
- Pinch ground cloves
- Pinch ground ginger
- Pinch ground allspice

Directions:

1. Combine all the ingredients in a slow cooker with a ceramic interior; set to low heat. Cover and cook overnight (for 8–9 hours). Stir and serve.

Nutrition Info: (Per Serving):Calories: 122; Total Fat: 1 g; Saturated Fat: 0 g; Cholesterol: 0 mg; Protein: 3 g; Sodium: 2 mg; Potassium: 262 mg; Fiber: 3 g; Carbohydrates: 26 g; Sugar: 10 g

Tofu Smoothie

Servings: 2

Ingredients:

- 1 cup frozen unsweetened peach slices
- 1 large banana, sliced
- 1/2 cup soft silken tofu
- 2 teaspoons honey
- 4 teaspoons toasted wheat germ
- Chilled water, as needed

Directions:

1. Put all the ingredients in a food processor or blender and process until smooth. Add a little chilled water, if necessary. Serve immediately.

Nutrition Info: (Per Serving):Calories: 166; Total Fat: 0 g; Saturated Fat: 0 g; Cholesterol: 0 mg; Protein: 6 g; Sodium: 10 mg; Potassium: 485 mg; Fiber: 4 g; Carbohydrates: 32 g; Sugar: 20 g

Breakfast Burritos

Servings: 6

Ingredients:

- 1 medium potato
- ½ pound (225 g) Sausage
- 1 small onion, chopped
- 1 teaspoon chili powder
- ¼ teaspoon cayenne pepper
- 2 eggs
- 6 flour tortillas
- 1 cup (110 g) Swiss cheese, shredded
- ¼ cup (45 g) tomato, chopped
- 2 tablespoons (30 g) sour cream
- ¼ cup (56 g) Dick's Best Salsa

Directions:

1. Cook potato in boiling water for 35 minutes until tender. When cool, peel and cut into cubes. Brown sausage in frying pan and add onion, chili powder, and cayenne pepper. Cook for 10 minutes. Drain and discard fat. Add cubed, cooked potato. Beat eggs and add to pan. Stir until eggs are set. Spoon mixture into center of warmed tortilla, top with

shredded cheese, and roll up tortilla to enclose mixture. For an authentic Mexican touch, serve topped with tomato, sour cream, and salsa.

Nutrition Info: (Per Serving): 132 g water; 443 calories (46% from fat, 18% from protein, 36% from carb); 19 g protein; 22 g total fat; 9 g saturated fat; 9 g monounsaturated fat; 2 g polyunsaturated fat; 40 g carb; 3 g fiber; 2 g sugar; 264 mg calcium; 3 mg iron; 306 mg sodium; 443 mg potassium; 616 IU vitamin A; 8 mg vitamin C; 131 mg cholesterol

Breakfast Tacos

Servings: 4

Ingredients:

- 4 eggs
- ¼ cup (56 g) Dick's Best Salsa
- ¼ cup (28 g) Swiss cheese, shredded
- 8 taco shells

Directions:

1. Scramble eggs, stirring in salsa and cheese when they are almost set. Divide into taco shells, sitting them upright in an 8 × 8-inch (20 × 20-cm) baking dish. Microwave for 1 minute or heat at 350°F (180°C, gas mark 4) for 5 minutes.

Nutrition Info: (Per Serving): 63 g water; 243 calories (51% from fat, 19% from protein, 30% from carb); 12 g protein; 14 g total fat; 4 g saturated fat; 5 g monounsaturated fat; 3 g polyunsaturated fat; 18 g carb; 2 g fiber; 1 g sugar; 142 mg calcium; 2 mg iron; 100 mg sodium; 165 mg potassium; 459 IU vitamin A; 2 mg vitamin C; 253 mg cholesterol

Baked French Toast

Servings: 6

Ingredients:

- 6 slices low sodium bread
- 3 eggs
- 3 tablespoons (39 g) sugar
- 1 teaspoon vanilla extract
- 2 ¼ cups (535 ml) skim milk
- ½ cup (60 g) all-purpose flour
- 6 tablespoons (90 g) brown sugar
- ½ teaspoon ground cinnamon, packed
- ¼ cup (55 g) unsalted butter
- 1 cup (145 g) blueberries, fresh or frozen

Directions:

1. Cut bread into 1-inch (2.5 cm)-thick slices and place in a greased 9 × 13-inch (23 × 33-cm) baking dish. In a medium bowl, lightly Beat eggs, sugar, and vanilla. Stir in the milk until well blended. Pour over bread, turning pieces to coat well. Cover and refrigerate overnight. Preheat oven to 375°F (190°C, gas mark 5). In a small bowl, Combine the flour, brown sugar, and cinnamon. Cut in butter

until mixture resembles coarse crumbs. Turn bread over in baking dish. Scatter blueberries over bread. Sprinkle evenly with crumb mixture. Bake for about 40 minutes until golden brown.

Nutrition Info: (Per Serving): 157 g water; 423 calories (27% from fat, 12% from protein, 61% from carb); 12 g protein; 13 g total fat; 6 g saturated fat; 4 g monounsaturated fat; 1 g polyunsaturated fat; 65 g carb; 2 g fiber; 31 g sugar; 216 mg calcium; 3 mg iron; 115 mg sodium; 341 mg potassium; 581 IU vitamin A; 2 mg vitamin C; 145 mg cholesterol

Blueberry-stuffed French Toast

Servings: 6

Ingredients:

- 3/4 cup mascarpone cheese
- 3 tablespoons powdered sugar
- 1/2 teaspoon grated lemon zest
- 12 slices French Bread , sliced 1" thick on a diagonal
- 1 cup fresh blueberries
- 1 cup milk
- 3 large eggs, beaten
- 2 tablespoons unsalted butter, melted
- 11/2 teaspoons vanilla

Directions:

1. In medium bowl, combine mascarpone cheese, powdered sugar, and lemon zest and mix well.
2. Place bread on work surface. Spread half of the slices with the cheese mixture and top with the blueberries, dividing evenly. Place remaining slices of bread on top and press together slightly to make sandwiches.

3. Arrange the bread sandwiches in a 13" × 9" glass baking dish.
4. In small bowl, combine milk, eggs, melted butter, and vanilla and beat until smooth. Pour into baking dish over bread.
5. Cover and refrigerate overnight.
6. In the morning, preheat the oven to 350°F. Uncover the baking dish and bake for 30–40 minutes or until tops of bread are golden brown. Serve immediately with maple syrup and more fresh blueberries.

Nutrition Info: (Per Serving):Calories: 398; Total Fat: 20 g; Saturated Fat: 20 g; Cholesterol: 153 mg; Protein: 11 g; Sodium: 116 mg; Potassium: 176 mg; Fiber: 2 g; Carbohydrates: 41 g; Sugar: 8 g

Fried Rice

Servings: 4

Ingredients:

- 3 tablespoons safflower or peanut oil, divided
- 1/2 cup minced cremini mushrooms
- 1 medium onion, chopped
- 2 cloves garlic, minced
- 1 tablespoon minced fresh ginger root
- 1 teaspoon five-spice powder
- 3 cups cold cooked white rice
- 2 large eggs, beaten
- 1/3 cup Vegetable Broth
- 1 cup frozen peas, thawed
- 1 tablespoon sesame oil

Directions:

1. In wok or large skillet, heat 1 tablespoon oil. Add the mushrooms; cook over low heat, stirring frequently, until the mushrooms are deep brown. Remove from wok and set aside.
2. Add remaining 2 tablespoons oil to wok. Stir-fry the onion, garlic, and ginger root until crisp-tender, about 5 minutes.

3. Sprinkle the food with the five-spice powder
    and add the rice to the wok; stir-fry until the
    rice is hot and slightly toasted.

4. Add the beaten eggs; stir-fry until the eggs
    are cooked and broken into small pieces. Add
    the vegetable broth, peas, mushrooms, and
    sesame oil; stir-fry until hot and serve
    immediately.

Nutrition Info: (Per Serving):Calories: 335; Total Fat: 16 g; Saturated Fat: 2 g; Cholesterol: 105 mg; Protein: 9 g; Sodium: 48 mg; Potassium: 297 mg; Fiber: 2 g; Carbohydrates: 37 g; Sugar: 2 g

Black Bean Chili

Servings: 6

Ingredients:

- 2 tablespoons safflower or peanut oil
- 2 medium onions, chopped
- 3 cloves garlic, minced
- 1 jalapeño pepper, minced
- 3 (14-ounce) cans no-salt-added black beans, rinsed and drained
- 2 (14-ounce) cans no-salt-added diced tomatoes, undrained
- 1 cup Spicy Salsa
- 1 tablespoon chili powder
- 1 teaspoon ground cumin
- 1 teaspoon smoked paprika
- 1 teaspoon dried oregano leaves
- 1/2 cup sour cream

Directions:

1. In medium saucepan, heat oil over medium heat. Add onions and garlic; cook and stir until tender, about 6 minutes. Place in 4- to 5-quart slow cooker.

2.   Add jalapeño, beans, tomatoes, and salsa to the slow cooker and stir well. Add chili powder, cumin, paprika, and oregano and stir.

3.   Cover and cook on low for 7–9 hours or until chili is bubbling. Serve topped with the sour cream.

Nutrition Info: (Per Serving):Calories: 133; Total Fat: 9 g; Saturated Fat: 2 g; Cholesterol: 10 mg; Protein: 3 g; Sodium: 49 mg; Potassium: 439 mg; Fiber: 3 g; Carbohydrates: 12 g; Sugar: 6 g

Sloppy Tofu Sandwiches With Zippy Coleslaw

Servings: 4

Ingredients:

- 1 (12-ounce) package firm tofu
- 2 tablespoons olive oil
- 1 medium onion, chopped
- 2 cloves garlic, sliced
- 1 cup chopped mushrooms
- 2 tablespoons no-salt-added tomato paste
- 1/2 cup Easy Homemade Ketchup
- 1/4 cup Mustard
- 1/4 cup water
- 2 tablespoons lemon juice
- 2 tablespoons brown sugar
- 1/8 teaspoon pepper
- 4 Hamburger Buns , split and toasted
- 11/2 cups Zippy Coleslaw

Directions:

1. Remove tofu from package and drain. Place tofu between layers of paper towel and press down firmly to remove water. Crumble the tofu coarsely.

102

2.   Heat olive oil in large nonstick pan over medium heat. Add onion, garlic, and mushrooms; cook until mushrooms give up their liquid and the liquid evaporates.

3.   Add tofu; cook, stirring frequently, until tofu and vegetables start to brown, about 8–9 minutes.

4.   Add tomato paste to pan; let brown in a few spots. Then stir in the ketchup, mustard, water, lemon juice, brown sugar, and pepper. Simmer for 5 minutes, stirring frequently.

5.   Make sandwiches with the hamburger buns, tofu mixture, and slaw.

Nutrition Info: (Per Serving):Calories: 629; Total Fat: 30 g; Saturated Fat: 5 g; Cholesterol: 40 mg; Protein: 18 g; Sodium: 20 mg; Potassium: 626 mg; Fiber: 6 g; Carbohydrates: 73 g; Sugar: 24 g

Sweet Potato Frittata

Servings: 8

Ingredients:

- 2 tablespoons olive oil
- 1 leek, chopped
- 1 large sweet potato, peeled and cubed
- 2 cloves garlic, minced
- 9 large eggs
- 1/4 cup light cream
- 1 tablespoon minced fresh thyme leaves
- 1/8 teaspoon pepper
- 1/3 cup shredded mozzarella cheese

Directions:

1. In 10" nonstick ovenproof skillet, heat olive oil over medium heat. Add leek and sweet potato. Cook, stirring frequently, until vegetables soften and start to turn brown, about 10–12 minutes. When they are tender, add the garlic and cook for 1 minute longer.

2. In large bowl, beat eggs with cream, thyme, and pepper. Add to skillet.

3. Cook the frittata over medium heat, lifting edges so uncooked egg flows underneath,

104

until the bottom is golden and edges are puffy, about 8–10 minutes.

4.   Preheat broiler. Top frittata with cheese and place 6" from heat source. Broil for 9–10 minutes, watching carefully, until the top is golden and the frittata is puffed. Serve immediately.

Nutrition Info: (Per Serving):Calories: 168; Total Fat: 12 g; Saturated Fat: 4 g; Cholesterol: 249 mg; Protein: 8 g; Sodium: 117 mg; Potassium: 154 mg; Fiber: 0 g; Carbohydrates: 6 g; Sugar: 2 g

Cauliflower Patties With Corn Compote

Servings: 4

Ingredients:

- 1 tablespoon olive oil
- 2 cups frozen corn kernels, thawed and drained
- 1 medium red bell pepper, chopped
- 2 cloves garlic, sliced
- 1 medium tomato, seeded and chopped
- 1 head cauliflower
- 2 large eggs
- 1/4 cup ricotta cheese
- 1/3 cup shredded Swiss cheese
- 2 tablespoons grated Parmesan cheese
- 2 slices French Bread , crumbled
- 1/2 teaspoon dried dill weed
- 1/8 teaspoon black pepper
- 2 tablespoons unsalted butter

Directions:

1. In medium skillet, heat olive oil over medium heat. Add corn, bell pepper, and garlic; cook, stirring occasionally, until tender, about 5

minutes. Add tomato; cook for another 3 minutes. Remove from heat and set aside.

2.   Cut the florets off the cauliflower and place in a microwave-safe dish. Peel the stems and chop into 1" pieces; add to florets in dish. Add water; cover and microwave for 8 minutes or until cauliflower is tender. Drain well.

3.   Transfer cauliflower to bowl and coarsely mash. Stir in eggs, ricotta, Swiss cheese, Parmesan cheese, bread crumbs, dill weed, and pepper; mix well. Form into 8 patties.

4.   Heat butter in large nonstick skillet over medium heat. Add the patties and cook in the butter, turning once, until golden brown, about 7–8 minutes total.

5.   Place patties on a serving plate and top with the corn mixture.

Nutrition Info: (Per Serving):Calories: 336; Total Fat: 118 g; Saturated Fat: 8 g; Cholesterol: 139 mg; Protein: 14 g; Sodium: 140 mg; Potassium: 482 mg; Fiber: 5 g; Carbohydrates: 33 g; Sugar: 7 g

Spanako-pitas

Servings: 4–6

Ingredients:

- 4 Pita Breads , cut in half
- 1 tablespoon extra-virgin olive oil
- 1 tablespoon unsalted butter
- 1 medium onion, chopped
- 3 cloves garlic, minced
- 3 tablespoons lemon juice, divided
- 4 cups baby spinach leaves
- 1/2 cup chopped flat-leaf parsley
- 2 tablespoons chopped fresh mint leaves
- 3 hard-cooked eggs, chopped
- 1/2 cup ricotta cheese
- 2 tablespoons crumbled feta cheese
- 1/2 teaspoon grated lemon zest

Directions:

1. Prepare the pita breads, cool, and cut in half crosswise. Open the pocket in the center, then set aside.
2. In medium saucepan, heat olive oil and butter over medium heat. Add onion and garlic; cook and stir until the onion starts to

108

turn golden around the edges, about 8–10 minutes. Remove from heat and stir in 2 tablespoons lemon juice.

3. Meanwhile, combine spinach, parsley, and mint in large bowl. Add the hot onion mixture and toss to coat; the spinach will wilt slightly. Add eggs and toss.

4. In small bowl, combine ricotta, feta, remaining 1 tablespoon lemon juice, and lemon zest and mix well. Spread this mixture inside the pita breads.

5. Add the spinach mixture to the pita breads and serve immediately.

Nutrition Info: (Per Serving):Calories: 252; Total Fat: 13 g; Saturated Fat: 5 g; Cholesterol: 125 mg; Protein: 10 g; Sodium: 130 mg; Potassium: 232 mg; Fiber: 2 g; Carbohydrates: 23 g; Sugar: 1 g

Lightning Source UK Ltd.
Milton Keynes UK
UKHW021102220721
387582UK00001B/38